DIET COOKBOOK FOR RHEUMATOID ARTHRITIS

A COMPLETE MEAL PLAN FOR RHEUMATOID ARTHRITIS

JOSH HAGGARD

Table of Contents

CHAPTER ONE

The diet for Rheumatoid Arthritis

Anyone can get rheumatoid arthritis (RA). Osteoarthritis, on the other hand, is caused by the gradual degeneration of joints over time. RA is caused by the body's own immune system attacking the joints in the body. The root cause of the problem is unknown. Painful swelling, stiffness, and inflammation ensue as a result, however.

This swelling and pain may be alleviated by consuming foods that reduce inflammation throughout your entire body. Of the 217 people with longstanding RA surveyed in 2017, 24% said that their RA symptoms were influenced by food in some way, either positively or negatively.

One way people with RA choose to support their health is by changing their diet. In conjunction with medical treatments such as over-the-counter painkillers, anti-inflammatory medications, and immune-suppressing therapies, certain foods may help you manage your RA symptoms.

An overview of foods to eat and avoid, as well as specific diets that may help people with RA live healthier lives, is provided below.

What to eat if you have RA? Here are some ideas.

Inflammatory symptoms may be alleviated by anti-inflammatory foods. Inflammation in the body is reduced by them. This effect can be attributed to a variety of different nutrients, ingredients, or other elements.

Antioxidants

RA disease activity may be improved by antioxidants. An over-production of reactive oxygen species (ROS) in your body can be eliminated by using these compounds. Inflammation can also be reduced by using them.

Foods rich in vitamins A, C, or E, as well as selenium, can help you get more of these nutrients. Green tea or fresh fruit and vegetable juices are both good options, as are both.

Fiber

Weight loss and a healthier gut microbiome are both possible benefits of dietary fiber. Increasing your intake of the following foods will help you get more fiber into your diet:

Produce that has been picked recently

• whole grain

• beans

• nuts

Flavonoids

Plants produce flavonoids, which are chemical compounds. When we eat fruits and vegetables, they find their way into our diets. Flavonoids have the ability to reduce inflammation in the body, which in turn can lessen the discomfort and swelling associated with RA. Flavonoids-rich foods include:

• berries

• a cup of green tea

• grapes

• broccoli

• soy

• semi-sweet chocolate

Spices

The anti-inflammatory properties of spices have long been known. Compound curcumin in turmeric has anti-inflammatory effects. Similar to ginger, it may have anti-inflammatory properties.

Curcumin, on the other hand, is less effective in the absence of piperine, a compound found in black pepper. In order to reduce inflammation, combine turmeric with a pinch of black pepper. Chili peppers contain a compound called capsaicin, which has anti-inflammatory properties.

A list of foods to avoid in the case of RA

It's best to eat anti-inflammatory foods while avoiding foods with a variety of common ingredients.

The following are some foods that may cause an inflammatory reaction:

• White flour and white sugar are examples of refined carbohydrates.

trans fatty acids, which can be found in fried foods;

Processed and red meats

• dairy

• eggs

If you're unable to avoid these foods entirely, eat fewer of them instead. Even a minor adjustment can have a positive impact on your RA symptoms. A good example of this is choosing fish instead of red meat, which is a common pro-inflammatory food swap.

Dietary guidelines from the Mediterranean region.

Anti-inflammatory foods are abundant in some diets. A good example of this is the Mediterranean diet. For arthritis sufferers, this diet is recommended by the Arthritis Foundation because it can help reduce inflammation.

Produce that has been picked recently

- fish

Pistachios and other tree nuts

- beans

- whole grain

oleocanthal

The Paleo diet is a way of eating that is based on the

Foods that our forebears would have eaten in the "old stone age" are the focus of the Paleo diet. It encourages the consumption of fruits and vegetables, which have been shown to reduce inflammation. However, there is a lot of red meat in there, which may have the opposite effect on weight loss. Before embarking on this diet, consult with your doctor.

* meat

- vegetables

- fruits

This diet is high in protein and low in carbohydrates, like many others. Additionally, Paleo diets do not include any grains, legumes, or dairy products.

- man-made food crops

- sugars

- dairy

- Foods prepared in a factory

There are health benefits to following a paleo diet, but only if you eat the right foods and aren't depriving yourself of anything you absolutely must. Discuss the paleo diet with your doctor to see if it is right for you.

If you want to reduce inflammation in your body, you may want to eat a more balanced, natural diet that is less restrictive of macronutrients.

The takeaway is

Rheumatoid arthritis (RA) is an autoimmune disease. Many people who have had RA for a long time have found that certain foods help or worsen their symptoms. This suggests that diet may play a role in the treatment of RA.

The Mediterranean diet, which emphasizes anti-inflammatory foods, may help alleviate the symptoms of RA. Inflammation can be exacerbated by foods that are known to cause it. People with rheumatoid arthritis (RA) can improve their health and well-being by making healthy food choices.

10 Foods to Help Reduce Inflammation in Rheumatoid Arthritis

Rheumatoid arthritis' most debilitating symptoms—pain, stiffness, and swelling—are all caused by inflammation. What should I do next? Your diet may play a role in the answer.

Rheumatoid arthritis (RA) patients had significantly more pro-inflammatory diets, according to research published in Arthritis Research & Therapy in April 2021. Those with RA who were able to reduce diet-associated inflammation between 2011 and 2017 also managed to maintain low disease activity. Study coauthor and director of the Cancer Prevention and Control Program at the University of South Carolina in Columbia, James R. Hébert, MSPH, ScD, said, "That particular result was extraordinarily strong and consistent as indicated by more than 3.5 times greater odds of maintaining good control over the disease in comparison with those who did not adopt a more anti-inflammatory diet."

Even more importantly, the long-term benefits of a low-inflammatory diet were demonstrated in this study, which was conducted over a period of several years. When it comes to long-term weight loss, "such a diet can be extraordinarily diverse and sensually pleasing," says Hébert, "it can be very easy to maintain."

CHAPTER THREE

A diet high in polyunsaturated fatty acids and plant fiber, such as omega-3 fatty acids and lots of fruits and vegetables, may reduce the risk of RA, according to additional research Fiber and polyunsaturated fatty acids are also thought to reduce levels of C-reactive protein (CRP), which is a marker of inflammation in the joints.

It's possible that phytonutrients found in fiber-rich fruits, vegetables, and grains may help alleviate some of the health benefits of fiber. The consumption of fish high in omega-3s, such as salmon and herring and mackerel, may also help reduce joint swelliness and tenderness, according to research.

Are There Foods That Are Safe for People With Joint Problems?

More research is needed to determine exactly how much of the compounds found in various foods can help alleviate the symptoms of RA.

The Western diet, with its emphasis on fast, cheap, and flavorful foods, is thought to be a contributing factor to the prevalence of autoimmune diseases like rheumatoid arthritis (RA).

For starters, obesity is definitely associated with inflammatory diseases. Increased levels of body fat lead to an increase in inflammatory substances in the body. Eating a lot of processed foods and fattening foods like fast food and fried food can increase inflammation.

Researchers are also learning more about the role that intestinal bacterial imbalances caused by a high-fat, low-nutrient diet may play in the development of such diseases and disorders.

It's possible that changing your diet may not reduce inflammation enough to warrant the abandonment of other RA management treatments, however. However, according to Lona Sandon, PhD, RDN, an associate professor in the department of clinical nutrition at the University of Texas

Southwestern Medical Center in Dallas and a RA patient herself, it can help reduce medication requirements and side effects. And, as Dr. Sandon points out, it's never been proven that eating well makes anything worse.

Discover which foods can help alleviate your symptoms and keep you healthy in the following paragraphs.

1

Olive oil may function similarly to NSAIDs in some ways.

The traditional Mediterranean diet, which is high in olive oil, has been linked to a lower incidence of inflammation-related diseases like degenerative joint disease and diabetes, prompting researchers to investigate the oil's anti-inflammatory properties.

Because it appears to suppress pain in the same way that nonsteroidal anti-inflammatory drugs (NSAIDS) like ibuprofen do, researchers have found that oleocanthal, an olive oil compound, is a useful pain reliever when used in cooking or salad dressings as part of a daily pain management regimen.

2

Vitamin C Is Essential for the Repair of Damaged Tissue.

According to Sandon, vitamin C is essential for the synthesis of collagen, which aids in the development and repair of blood vessels, tendons, ligaments, and bone.

As a general rule, the current recommended daily allowance for vitamin C in the United States is 75 milligrams (mg) for women and 90 mg for men. Aim for 85 mg if you're pregnant, and for lactating women, aim for 120 mg.

Aside from their abundant supply of anti-inflammatories

and vitamins C and B1, these citrus fruits and vegetables are also good sources of fiber, which is helpful for people with rheumatoid arthritis. Oral cyclosporine and methotrexate, two common RA medications, may be affected by citrus's ability to pass through the body unhindered. Other studies suggest that other citrus juices, like those made from Seville oranges, limes, and pomelos, may also affect how CYP3A4 works in the body. Regular consumption of grapefruit juice blocks the protein known as

CYP3A4 that helps the body metabolize cyclosporine.

It's possible to get vitamin C from other sources like tomatoes, peppers, melons, strawberries, kiwi or potatoes if you're taking medications that can be affected by citrus. There is a significant amount of vitamin C in a half-cup cooked broccoli.

Avoiding citrus juices while taking your medication is another option, advises Sandon. It's better to eat citrus fruits or juices at a different time of the day. Talk to your doctor about the best diet and medication regimen for you.

3

Antioxidants and Inflammation-Fighting Capabilities in Berries

One or more servings of fresh or frozen blueberries, raspberries, strawberries, or blackberries should be part of your daily diet according to Sandon's recommendation. They contain powerful antioxidants, such as proanthocyanins and ellagic acid, which combat inflammation and cell damage by reducing oxidative stress in the body. According to Sandon, the amount and composition of the compounds differ depending on the type of berry.

4

The Beta-Carotene and Vitamin A found in carrots may help reduce the symptoms of arthritis.

CHAPTER FOUR

Sandon recommends including anti-arthritis foods like carrots, squash, and sweet potatoes on your shopping list. Vitamin A and beta-carotene, which are abundant in these and other orange-hued vegetables, are thought to combat inflammation. These compounds are more readily available when they are heated up in the kitchen. Eating these vegetables in recommended serving sizes on a regular basis will provide the greatest health benefits, as will consuming them in large quantities. About one large carrot, or seven to ten small ones, makes up a half-cup serving of carrots.

5

A Diet Rich in Whole Grains May Help You Lose Weight and Relieve Pain.

Whole grains have gotten a lot of press lately, and for good reason, according to Sandon. Whole grains are those that retain the bran (the outer hull), endosperm, and germ of the original grain.

Compared to refined grains, whole grains provide more fiber and essential nutrients like selenium, potassium, and magnesium. As an added benefit, studies show that a diet high in whole grains helps people with RA maintain better weight control.

Sandon recommends switching to whole wheat bread and whole grain pasta. Caution: Beware of misleading labels on whole wheat bread. The Oldways

Whole Grain Council's Whole Grain Stamp should indicate that it is made from 100% whole wheat. You can also include other whole grains in your diet, such as oatmeal for breakfast or a bulgur salad for dinner.

6

Spice up your food with ginger to bring down the heat.

Aspirin and ibuprofen-like anti-inflammatory drugs, such as

ginger, contain compounds that work in a similar way. The flavor of this multipurpose root is also noteworthy. Stir-fries, sushi, and acorn squash soup all benefit from the addition of fresh peeled ginger.

Sandon advises against taking ginger supplements without first consulting a physician about their ability to reduce inflammation. The thinning of the blood can be dangerous if you are taking Coumadin, for example, if you eat too much ginger (warfarin). In addition, it can cause hypoglycemia by lowering blood sugar levels. For those taking high blood pressure medication, ginger may have an effect on their blood pressure.

7

Pineapple's enzymes can reduce swelling, according to research.

Stocksy

According to Sandon, the enzyme bromelain, which is abundant in pineapple, has been linked to a reduction in osteoarthritis and rheumatoid arthritis pain and swelling. So, whenever possible, include this tropical fruit in your diet. For a sweet-and-sour flavor, try it in fruit salads, baked in savory dishes or incorporated into smoothies.

It is possible to buy Bromelain supplements, but it is advised that you consult your doctor first due to the possibility of increased bleeding when combined with blood thinners like Plavix (clopidogrel bisulphate), Coumadin, or aspirin. Antibiotics and sedatives may also be affected by bromelain's effects.

8

Adding Turmeric to Your Diet May Help Reduce Inflammation

Curcumin is a naturally occurring polyphenol found in the Indian spice turmeric. According to a study published in Food Chemical Toxicology in September 2015, curcumin has antioxidant and anti-inflammatory properties. While it's still unclear exactly how much of it is required to have a positive impact, why not experiment with it in your cooking to see if it makes a difference?

9

Indulge Your Sore Joints With A Cup Of Green Tea

The catechins in green tea help to halt the production of inflammation. "The consumption of green tea offers an overall anti-inflammatory effect," according to a study published in Toxicology and Applied Pharmacology in August 2017. Most studies have relied on small populations. "Real-world, large-scale study" was the focus of a study published in the Annals of Nutrition and Metabolism on March 20, 2020. Increased green tea consumption was linked to lower disease activity in the study.

10

Antioxidants may be boosted by drinking cherry juice.

According to a study published in the Journal of Functional Foods, drinking Montmorency tart cherry juice lowers uric acid levels and boosts blood levels of antioxidants called anthocyanins. In any case, Sandon cautions, don't take this news too seriously just yet. Despite the fact that cherry juice is a healthy food in moderation, more research is needed to determine how much one should drink to reap the benefits. Be adventurous and try it with seltzer instead of sodas!

THE END

www.ingramcontent.com/pod-product-compliance
Lightning Source LLC
Chambersburg PA
CBHW051403150726
48000CB00003B/1318